F.B.I. WARNING
Copyrighted Material

I0429919

Vision
Is
Possible

Improve Your Vision and get a Facelift for Free!

An original vision program targeting your Eye Lids.

Jumper Publications and Media
from Advice to Results

Disclaimer

The purpose of this book is to empower the reader with knowledge, to educate, informational purposes. This book is not medical advice, but rather the author's personal experience, and is a guide for anyone who wishes to implement said dietary or lifestyle changes at the reader's own discretion. The choice between medical care and self care is completely up to the reader. If you have a medical problem, seek medical care. The author and Jumper Publications and Media shall not be held responsible or liable for any and all damages, loss, or injury, of any kind that may be caused or allegedly caused, directly or indirectly, by the information in this book. Reading beyond this page is the reader's consent to the above disclaimer.

Other Publications

ABC Water and the Number Crunch Diet
a step by step solution to alkaline deficiency and
with a New and Unique approach to weight control

Nontoxic Teeth Whitening and Dental Hygiene System
"Spare me the chemicals, I've switched to FOOD GRADE to
whiten, gargle and brush."

JPM Oral Hygiene Protocol
stop using toxic drugstore mouthwash, discover how to reduce
your gum pocket depth from 3-4-3 to 1-2-1 mm when they probe

12 Changes A Year – Volume 1
the recipe book to the Number Crunch Diet
When you take control of the numbers
you take control of your weight.

NCD Flaxseed Shake Recipe
the Number Crunch Diet method for getting omega 3s
and with three variations so you'll never get bored

The 5 Points of Posture
the missing link to fat loss, overall wellness, and
to becoming Respected, Adored, and Wealthy

12 Changes A Year – Volume 2
the recipe book to the Number Crunch Diet
Begin today and forever be in control of the numbers you're eating.

To purchase additional copies, please visit

http://www.CreateSpace.com/5000428

CONTENTS

Edits & Format

You will notice oddities in punctuation, spelling, syntax, and perhaps even semantics, within this book. Feel free to let me know, but some of it is done for brevity or to shift emphasis. I use capitals where I see fit, to grab your attention and make it stand out, and I also remove capitals when I don't think they are deserving of them, or to remove emphasis after first usage, i.e., Pyrex becomes pyrex. And french bread, brussels sprouts, and english cucumbers, are spelled lowercase, as we are not going to "link" a European vacation to our food and eating.

Secondly, I will unhyphenated to create rhythm. Grammatically, two or more words that function as an adjective before a noun are supposed to be hyphenated. That's fine. A million-dollar smile, is the adjective "million-dollar" describing the smile. However, this can get redundant after a while, 1&2 3, 1&2 3, 1&2 3. The noun gets all the attention. But what if you want the adjectives to have the emphasis? After all, the adjectives are the descriptive words. So, I will drop the hyphens to allow the adjectives equal emphasis, and to change the pace of the sentence a bit. So if there are no hyphens, read it slower and evenly, one two three four five six seven. A "step-by-step solution" sounds a bit skippy and simplistic, whereas, a "step by step solution" is said slower and sounds more methodical. Hyphenating two words, or joining two words as a compound word, reduces their individual meanings.

With regard to fastfood, healthfood, and seasalt, it's time for these words to evolve into compound words, so the trend starts here.

There are also some fragmented sentences, subject-verb disagreements, and singular/plural violations. When "correcting" certain of these sentences, they lost their emphasis and punch, so I kept them as is.

In the past I've been guilty of judging other author's sentences, only to reread it with the commas, pauses, and then it made perfect sense. So, if there's a comma, then pause, as you may not get to pause later in the sentence. If there's no comma, then don't pause and read it all as one.

I pose questions, but without question marks. Some are rhetorical, but some are to make you Ponder. Great word. Ponder. If you see a question mark at the end, then it requires an answer. If there's no question mark, then you can just say, yeah, no, or hm.

English continues to change, people using it, customize the language to fit what they want to communicate, emphasize, and to make their point from various angles. It also has to have a variety of melodies and rhythms to keep it from being boring. If you find yourself having to reread a sentence, it may be that it's structured that way for that very reason. So take your time. Don't rush. Let the words digest, so that you absorb the material, and hopefully take some of it and make it a part of your life.

Lastly, you will notice that I customized the headers of every page! This is not something Microsoft Word Starter allows you to do. You can only customize three pages, first, even, and odd. So, to get around this I had to create a Page Break every three pages, and as a result, the last line of some of the pages doesn't "justify" to the edge. So I hope that flipping through the upper corners of the pages will assist you in finding the chapter that you are looking for.

You won't see any citations from scientific studies or PubMed, because at JPM we look to a higher source for our reference.

God Bless!

Enjoy the Journey

Email me if you have a question, or if you just want to comment. Your purchase comes with 3-months free support and photos.

Barry Ogston, B.Sc., CLS, MLS(ASCP)

You have to crunch the numbers to see what you're really eating.

CHAPTER 1

Introduction

Hi! And Welcome!

Of all the publications published by JPM, this one is likely to be the least impressive. You are free to try vision supplements or vision focusing programs. I've tried them. All I can say is, I wasn't fully satisfied with the results. So, I came up with my own exercises. I am also a big believer in plant colors and eating them. See the *Number Crunch Diet* and *12 Changes a Year* for ways to add plant colors to your diet. Clearly, bad diet => bad vision, and, good diet => good vision. Let food be thy medicine – Hippocrates.

The vision exercise book and program that I purchased was *Rebuild Your Vision*, by Orlin G. Sorensen. Great program for the eyeball and ocular muscles, but almost nothing with regard to eyelids. And let's face it, tired eyes and droopy eyelids result in diminished vision. The exercises in *Rebuild Your Vision* do work, and help, but if you need more, like I did, then add eyelid exercises. His book and program is a bit expensive, I think I paid $100, but look on the internet and maybe you can find eyeball and eye focusing exercises for free. If money is not a problem, buy the program and read it and do the exercises. $100 is a small price to pay for better vision and ocular muscle awareness.

So the exercises that I've come up with are very "specific". So, forgive me if this booklet is overly detailed and dry-ish. However, if you really take the information and use it, if your experience is like mine, you will find your vision will improve, your eyes will look brighter, and your face and eye area will look younger. I do these exercises every day, several times a day. In fact, the VIP exercises are the only ones I do, and I only rarely do the eye focusing exercises from RYV.

The other methods, vitamins and minerals, and eye focusing exercises, do have their place, so I encourage you to explore them. But if you find it's not enough, or not really doing anything, then try adding-in the exercises that follow. So let's begin!

CHAPTER 2

JPM Eyelid Stretch™

Double Brow Lift – again, if you are wanting eyeball exercises, this is not the book, or if you want to take bilberry or drink carrot juice, by all means go-for-it, but this book is 'Outer' Eye, lids and brows.

Step 1
Lift your eyebrows to the ceiling. Up as high as you can. Try to isolate just the eyebrows. Now relax, and drop back to normal. Do ten of these. The tempo is "one second up" "one second down" "one second up" "one second down", eight more times.

Now repeat this exercise with two seconds up and two seconds down. Say, "Up Up" "Down Down", or, "Up Hold" "Down Hold", ten times. Up Hold Down Hold = 1

Step 2
Now, lift both brows and hold. Now, close your eyes but keep your brows reaching for the ceiling. Now, press your eyelids down hard while reaching for the ceiling with your brows, BUT, no squinting. Don't do "squinting eyes" or create wrinkles, aka, "crow's feet". Just do two things, brows to the ceiling, lids down to the floor. So, you have the JPM Eye Lid Stretch™.

Hold this position, like how you would hold any muscle stretch, and become aware of how it feels. Is there fatigue? Does one side feel fresh but the other side feels tender?

Hold this for a count of ten. You don't have to be "religious" about the count of ten, but rather, just feel the stretch, become aware of any fatigue or soreness, and then open and relax.

I do this Eyelid Stretch several times a day. You can do it at the computer, while sitting at a stoplight while driving, anywhere. It takes ten seconds, so if you don't do this several times a day, or at least once or twice a day, then you are not serious about improving your surrounding-eye muscles and vision.

On the contrary, once you begin doing this you will find it totally freshens your eyes and face. It's like pressing the "refresh" key on your computer.

Now, in the stretch position, with the brows up and the lids pressing down, move your eyeball around. Just simple side to side, and up and down. Nothing intense. Just keep the brows up high to the ceiling and the lids closed and pressing down. Notice freshness or fatigue. Just gently move the eyeball around in various directions to stretch-out the fatigue. Then rest.

Don't make the stretching intense. Keep it mild. If you feel fatigue, then do the exercise again in 1-2 hours, i.e., several times a day.

It's better to keep it mild and do it several times a day.

Single Eyelid Stretch
Now, with both of your brows lifted to the ceiling, close just the left eyelid. Basically, just do the same stretch, eyelid down, BUT, the right one stays open. Don't squint the eye, like when you "wink". Just do two things, both brows up, left lid down.

Hold.

Get comfortable with that. Some people may not be able to do it. Don't worry. Keep trying it. I couldn't do my right side in the beginning but now I have no problems doing it on either side.

Now, watch yourself in the mirror as you do this Left Lid Stretch, or left lid blink. You should see only ONE thing moving, your left eyelid. Check yourself in the mirror and try to isolate just the left eyelid. Only one thing should be happening, the left eyelid comes down, hold, and comes up.

Try that and get comfortable with it.

Now, once you have that down. Do it again, BUT, look at your right eye as you do it. That means, both brows are up, and you bring just your left lid down, and hold. Look in the mirror at your RIGHT eyelid. Is it fully open? It should be fully open. Unfortunately, what happens when we close just the left eyelid, we also close the right one a little bit.

Your goal is to blink with the left while keeping the right perfectly unmoved. So, both brows up, left lid comes down, right lid doesn't move.

I can do this perfectly on the left, but when I do it on the right, my left eyelid closes a bit. It's my weak spot. I'm still working at it.

Try this JPM Single Eyelid Blink™ on both sides. Blink just the left eyelid, while keeping the right eyelid wide open, fully open. Then do the other side. Both brows up, and blink the right lid, while keeping the left lid wide open.

I can blink my left eyelid and while watching my right side, the eyelid doesn't move at all. It's perfect. This is your goal.

So, even though you are blinking with the left, your concentration is on the right. Same is true for the other side. If you are blinking on the right, your concentration is on keeping the left eyelid completely open and don't allow it to move or close any.

This is quite hard to do on both sides. If you can get both sides perfect, that is, no movement of the other eyelid, the "nonworking eyelid", the nonblinking side, then you've mastered this exercise.

So, at first just try to blink, just the left, and then just the right. Then, once you've got that mastered on both sides, then work on keeping the "nonblinking" eyelid unmoved and completely open.

If your eye is completely open, as when you are doing the Double Brow Lift, the iris of the eye should be completely seen. The colored part of the eye, the iris, is a round circle, and you should be able to see the entire round circle of the iris when you blink right and left. So, when you blink the left lid, you should be able to see the full round circle of the right iris.

Try it on both sides. Right and Left blinking.

Do not squint, and do not lift or tense the lower eyelid.

Do not tighten the facial muscles or lift the cheeks or wink or any of that. Only do the two movements.
1. Both brows up to the ceiling.
2. Left lid down and hold, while keeping the right unmoved and completely open as you do so, so you can see the full circle of the iris.

This is a very effective exercise. I do this several times a day. My right-eye blink with the left eye fully open is getting better, but after a few tries, it gets tired and drops down a bit and covers the iris some. But it is much better than it once was. My left eye is my weak muscle side. Probably due to the wind drying out my left eye while driving with the car window open.

Again, if you do this a few times you will be worn out, tired, so it's better to do it a few times and check your progress in the mirror and then that's all for now. Do it again in an hour or two. And do it every day, several times a day. It works. In my experience.

Keeping your eyes fully open is, in my opinion, one reason for not having perfect vision. Your eyes aren't fully open! This will make your face look younger as well, the "facelift" part.

CHAPTER 3

The Flicker

Okay, we are going to do the advanced version of that exercise. I call it the Nora Desmond. How gay, I know. But if you've ever watched the *Carol Burnett Show* from the 1970s and 80s, you will recall a skit where Carol was Nora Desmond and Harvey Korman was Max, and she would slap him across the face and Harvey couldn't stop laughing on camera. Half the comedy was the fact that Harvey couldn't say his lines because he was always laughing.

Carol Burnett could move her eyebrows up, down, right side, left side, she could blink right side, left side. She was a master at isolating her eyes, eyelids, and eyebrows. So, in this skit, she would have one eye wide open and the other eye in the closed position, but only 90% closed and flickering, or twitching, vibrating. This is hard to do. Let's try it.

To begin, both brows up. Now, keeping the right eyelid unmoved and completely open, close the left eyelid, but flicker it and vibrate it at the bottom. Again, only two movements. Brows up. Left lid down and flicker it.

The lid is only 90% closed, 10% open, at the bottom. Unlike the previous exercise where we closed the eyelid and tried to press down to the floor, in this exercise we are not pushing the eyelid down. Just close the eyelid 90% of the way, letting it rest on the lower lid, and vibrate or flicker it, twitch it.

Then try the other side. Both brows up, right lid comes down, left lid stays unmoved and fully open, and with the right lid 95% closed, flicker it. Or 90% closed. Just not pressed-down closed.

Again, this is hard to do if you concentrate on the "nonblinking" eyelid and keeping it unmoved and fully open so you can see the entire circle of the iris.

I also do this a couple of times a day. If I've done the previous exercises, which I do first, then I may be too tired to do this "Nora Desmond". This is why it's better just to do 30-60 seconds of exercises and then do it several times a day. Don't worry if people think you're weird, they are likely wearing glasses, contacts, or candidates for surgery. Why not just do some eyelid exercises daily and avoid all that.

You can do the blinks from the previous chapter as follows.
1. Brows up
2. 10 blinks left, even tempo, down up down up down up, 7 more
3. 10 blinks right, even tempo

Next time do:
1. Brows up
2. 10 blinks left, slow tempo, down hold up hold, 9 more
3. 10 blinks right, slow tempo

Next time do:
1. Brows up
2. 10 blinks alternating, left right left right left right, 7 more

Next time do:
1. Brows up
2. 10 blinks alternating, slow, L-down L-up, R-down R-up, 8 more

Then repeat all four of these with the Nora Desmond, 90% closed blinks with the flicker at the bottom of each blink.

That would be eight times a day total. If you do this every day, even just 3-4 times a day for a few seconds, you will notice that you get better at it. It's tiring on your brain as well as your eyes as you have to create a mind-muscle connection. You might think that this is stupid, but it works. You can wear glasses and struggle with your vision, or you can build your eyelid muscles and open up your eyes more so you can see.

And if you did see Carol Burnett on TV, you will recall she had "eyes wide open", big wide open eyes. And, her face looked pretty good too as I recall. Or you can go to your cosmetic surgeon and pay $10,000 to have him tighten the sides of your face. Lucille Ball was another TV celebrity that had eyes wide open. And I don't recall either of these two ladies needing to wear glasses.

Chapter Endnote
Someone said that Carol had a facelift later in life, I don't know about that, but if she did, it wasn't from having weak surrounding-eye muscles. Being on stage requires putting on-and-off a lot of makeup. Performers who put a lot of makeup on-and-off, day-after-day, week-after-week, year-after-year, often end up with wrinkled skin later in life. It's the price they pay to entertain us. If you've ever seen a stage performer or celebrity without makeup, well you know what I mean. So, the wisdom here is, don't wear makeup and your skin won't wrinkle as you get older. Many "earthy" holistic women know this. But you can't assume that will be enough. You need exercise too! Let's Go!

CHAPTER 4

Brow Lifts

Okay, let's do ten Double Brow Lifts. Ready, Up Down Up Down Up Down Up Down, five, six, seven, eight, nine, ten. Good. Do this one time, a couple of times a day. Many people never do this, hence, a decade later, their eyes are looking older and smaller. Take a look at some of the old/older people on TV. Some of them, their eyes are barely even open, making them appear old. Gravity is pulling all of that down. So if you don't lift it up, how do you expect it to look young and fresh?

That question has a question mark. So you have to answer it. How do you expect your face and eyes to look lifted and open and young if you never lift them? They tell you to exercise your body, right? Well, that's to keep it in-shape and working and young. If your vision is lacking, there are many possible reasons, but one of them is because your surrounding-eye area, brows and lids, are weak.

Muscles lose strength as we age, that's just the process of life. So you have to work them.

Okay, ten more DBLs, let's go, ready, One, Two, Three, Four, Five, Six, Seven, Eight, Nine, Ten! Good. If you did them, good for you! If you read that and didn't do them, well, Jumper Publications are not for you. JPM is all about giving you practical ways to fix and help something – THEN YOU HAVE TO DO IT. It's "do-it-yourself" care, Selfcare, Do, Do it. Action=>Results

So this double brow lift x10 is so easy that everyone can do it. It is your starting-point exercise. Maybe you can't do the other exercises that well or at all, but this DBL can be done by everyone. Make it your "go-to" exercise. Start with this DBL and do ten reps (repetitions) several times a day. There's no excuse. You can do it anywhere.

Now we're going to isolate just the left brow. Just lift the left eyebrow. Try hard not to move any other parts. When I first started to do this, I could lift the left side but I was not isolating it, i.e., that is to say, as I lifted the left eyebrow, the right was also going up some. Now I can do the left side perfectly. I can lift my left eyebrow up and nothing else moves. So, with practice it is possible. My right side was completely void of any mind-muscle connection. I couldn't lift my right brow at all. Now I can though. It takes a while, and I still need to work on isolating just the right brow because other parts are moving on the lift.

You have to create a wrinkle in your forehead above the brow when you lift it. On the left, mine is good. But on the right side, my "forehead wrinkle" is a bit less.

To help get the feel of this, do winks. To lift the left brow, wink with the right eye. Your right brow will come down as you wink on the right, and your left brow should go up. Practice this SBL, Single Brow Lift, with the winks to build up strength and a mind-muscle connection, then omit the wink and just do the isolated single brow lift.

So,
Step 1 – DBL, double brow lifts
Step 2 – SBLwW, single brow lifts with Wink
Step 3 – SBL, single brow lift
Step 4 – SBL, single brow lift, perfectly isolated and high/big

Many many people never do any sort of lifting at all. And then the years go by and they find their eyes getting smaller and looking older and their vision's not as good and they rub their eyes because

11

their eyes are weak and more easily fatigued. If you're wealthy or on TV, you'll opt for eyebrow surgery to lift them up and make them younger. Or, if you don't get the surgery, you age, and the appearance of your eyes ages, and your vision ages.

Am I telling you the truth or am I telling you the truth? I'm telling you the truth. So for me, the solution is easy, just add-in a few eye exercises every day here-and-there sporadically for 30 seconds each time. How hard is that. Not hard at all. You just have to decide you're going to do it. And I'm certain you will!! ☺

Key things to remember are:
1. Don't do a lot at one time, just ten reps of an exercise, 30sec.
2. Isolate. Keep working at it until you can completely isolate it.

To help you picture the SEB, Single Eye Blink, where you start with both brows up to the ceiling, and then just blink the left, down and up. Then do the right, down and up. To help you think of this, picture those dolls, Marie Osmond used to sell dolls on the *QVC Network* channel, and one of the dolls had eyelids that you could move up and down. So, imagine you want to close and open your left eyelid just like that doll. Nothing else moves except the eyelid. Close and Open. Down and Up. Then do the right side. Close and Open . Down and Up. Nothing on the doll moves except the one eyelid. AND, the nonworking eye stays wide open and doesn't close down. The iris of the nonworking eye is a big round circle. Remember how we did that? As you blink with the left, you look at your right eye to see if it goes down a bit or if it stays wide open and unmoved. You want it to stay wide open and unmoved. The iris should be fully visible and seen.

If you can do the SEB, single eye blink, on both sides with the nonworking eye being completely wide open and unmoved, then you have mastered this exercise.

If you can do this, both sides, perfectly, and you are just reading this, well, you are the exception, and you are probably aware that most people, the vast majority of people, do not have that much isolated control over their eyelid muscles. Again, think of the doll and how it can close and open one eyelid with complete isolation of all the other parts. If you can do this on both sides, Wow! Your vision problem must be due to the eye itself and not the surrounding area. My suggestion to you is to keep-it-up, "use-it or lose-it", because as we age our mind-muscle connection and the muscles themselves fade without specific conscious use of them.

So, we have the following exercises.
1. SEB – 10 left, 10 right, even tempo, down up, 9 more
2. SEB – 10 left, 10 right, with a hold, down hold up hold
3. SEB – 10 alternating LRLRLR, 7 more
4. SEB – 10 alternating, slower, L-down L-up, R-down R-up

Repeat 1-4 with the flicker eyelid, 90-95% closed, 5-10% open.

And now we have,
1. DBL – 10 double brow lifts, your "go-to" exercise
2. DBL – 10 with a hold, up hold down hold, 9 more
3. SBL – 10 single brow lifts, up down, 9 more, then the other side
4. SBL – 10 with holds, up hold down hold, 9 more, other side
5. SBL – 10 with winking, 10 left side, 10 right side
6. SBL – 10 with winking, alternating RLRL, 8 more

Again, done with 100% isolation, "Marie Osmond doll" eyelids.

If you can do all that, then I would say, "You're right up there with Carol and Lucy! Ready for your own TV show!"

CHAPTER 5

JPM Night Vision Exercise™

This next one isn't hard to do, physically, but likely very hard to do if you're "caught up in the rat race" and always have to be doing something. For this exercise, you will wait a few hours after the sun has gone down, and find a dark room or garage or someplace where it's completely black, pitch-black dark, when you turn off the light. This may mean that you have to cover up a digital clock or unplug it, or cover little red lights on surge protectors or computers, or other things like that. If there are windows and street lights, that won't work. You will need to find some place that is completely dark.

You will also want to have some items in that room so that as your vision adjusts, you can begin to see the items. An empty closet won't work as there's nothing for you to look at. You will also need a timer, I use the Acurite big-digit timer, be sure it can "count down" from a set time. And you may want to have a chair, I stand.

JPM Night Vision Exercise™
Take your timer into your room, set it for 20 minutes, turn off the lights, everything should appear black and you can't see two-feet in front of you, nothing, completely black. Start your timer. After five minutes, or ten minutes, you should be able to see some things in the room. Try to focus on those things and try to see them better. Keep doing this until your timer goes off. At 20 minutes, look for the item in the room that just at that moment became

visible. That is your "20 minute item". For me, it's a book that is across the room from where I am standing. At 5 minutes I can see some things, it's not pitch-black anymore. At 10 minutes I can see more, about 50%. At 15 minutes it's looking pretty good, pretty clear, but not 100%. And at 20 minutes, I can see the book and everything clearly.

This book is my baseline. Tomorrow or the next day, do the exercise again. This time, as soon as you see the "book" stop your timer. The timer may say 00:15. If you set it for 20 minutes and press start, it will count down. So your new night-vision-adjustment time is now 19 minutes and 45 seconds. You've cut 15 seconds off of your "Night Vision Adjustment" time.

Try not to daydream or tune-out while you do this exercise, but rather, continue to look around the room from your standing point, or sitting point, and try to focus-in on things. Try to make your eyes see in the dark. Opening your eyes wide helps. So the previous exercises will work to help this exercise. As you stand there for 20 minutes, work your eyes the entire time. Look around the room. Try to see. Keep looking in the direction of your "20 minute item" to see if you can see it yet.

This exercise works. I can attest to that. I've cut my time in half. I no longer "freak out" because I can't see when the lights are off, as I know that my night vision will be up-and-running within a minute, and I will be seeing things in 2-3 minutes, and seeing most things in five minutes, and pretty much everything clearly in ten minutes. BUT, again, you have to work your eyes. It isn't just going to happen. You have to do the exercise.

How long will it take you, I can't say anything about you, and you know that, everyone's different. I can only tell you that it works if you do it. Do it. Do It Yourself, care. Selfcare!

Now, keep in mind that nutrition plays a big role in health. If you are lacking in nutrients, your body goes to make a new cell, and it can't find what it needs so it makes a 90% perfect cell, or an 80%

perfect cell, or maybe even a 50% perfect cell, a cell that's just 50% operable. For this, I recommend the Number Crunch Diet, and the recipes found in *12 Changes A Year*. Not only will you get control of your weight by getting control of the numbers you're eating, but it's a long-term way of eating that contains Complete Nutrition, Maximum Freedom, and Total Control.

So, nutrition. Your body won't work right if it's deficient in Good, and getting too much Bad.

You might think, carrot juice or copper or bilberry. Well, that's fine, but there are two essential "seek out" fats often overlooked. See the *NCD Flaxseed Shake Recipe*. Just read the front and back covers and you will sense that it's not like all the others out there.

Vision is not my area of expertise. Self-health Strategies is. *The 5 Points of Posture* can help you with your anxiety. "Become Grounded and Unmoved" and say good-bye to intimidation.

The alkalinity component to health is completely hidden from the masses, and yet every nurse, doctor, or clinical lab scientist is well aware of acidosis and death. It's the primary reason for ordering an Arterial Blood Gas test. They need to know the pH. The Oxygen Saturation, O_2 Sat, can be obtain from the pulse oximeter, pulse ox. All the numbers on an ABG panel are important and help to identify what's going on, but the pH number is the most important.

You can discover your alkaline status, just like how you can discover your blood-pressure status, by reading and following what's in the book, *ABC Water and the Number Crunch Diet* – a step by step solution to alkaline deficiency. Never mind alkaline foods, I explain why in the book. The goal is an alkaline BODY.

For ocular-muscle exercises, look on the web, or buy Orlin's *Rebuild Your Vision*. It's very good for ocular muscles and focusing exercises. Their company also sells a vision supplement, it's good. But for surrounding-eye exercises, I like the VIP!

PREVIEW
from the
ABC Water and the Number Crunch Diet

As you know, the recipes for the NCD are being published under the titles, *12 Changes a Year* – the companion guide to the Number Crunch Diet. It may take up to a year to get them written as it will comprise about three volumes. In the meantime, you can get your pH paper testing set up and determine your current alkaline stores. The recipes read like a book and include additional information that I've discovered about diet, lifestyle, health and selfcare. I look forward to seeing you over there!

To join my mission in providing people with safe, effective, affordable, selfcare protocols, send someone you know to www.abcwaterandthenumbercrunchdiet.com. Tell them to take the Quiz!! Thanks for your support! God Bless.

Jumper Publications & Media
From Advice to Results

I almost forgot! (again, not really) to tell you!

If you liked this shake recipe be sure to check out

TCY
12 Changes a Year
Vol 2

for the NCD ORANGE SHAKE!
It makes 9, and I often repeat the recipe midweek.
And whey protein – but not from powder.

BUY THE BOOK!!
IT'S GOOD STUFF!

Leave a Review

Without giving away the contents, "spoilers", recommend this publication and leave a review so that someone else might benefit from it too. Thank you.

www.amazon.com   Search: Vision Is Possible

Subscribe to my YouTube Channel
www.youtube.com   Search: Number Crunch Diet

Be sure to send me an email so I can periodically keep in touch with updates and new Selfcare Strategies – and discount offers on new items (yes, more than books!) (a simple and effective weight-loss device) (a weightlifting "device" that I use EVERY time I work out) and don't forget the recipes! – TCY.

abcwaterandthenumbercrunchdiet@mail.com
Privacy – your email address will not be used for anything other than by Jumper Publications and Media.

Saliva vs Urine pH

Top Ten Reasons Why Saliva pH Is Worthless When Compared To Urine pH For Acid-Base Analysis

#10 Small Volume – small tiny volume samples don't represent the whole

#9 Difficult to Obtain – the procedure is to bring up saliva and swallow, 2x, then use the third one for the test, too hard to obtain

#8 Poor Reproducibility – when you retest your saliva sample, you will likely get a slightly different color (reading)

#7 Poor Accuracy – if you collect a second sample, it will likely give you a different reading than the first

#6 Bacterial Contamination – bacteria from your mouth will interfere with the test

#5 Food Contamination – food from your mouth will interfere with the test

#4 Spoon Contamination – the surface of the spoon that you collect it on is going to affect your small sample

#3 Viscosity – saliva is too thick and results in faded or dual colors of the test pad (or paper)

#2 Difficulty Reading – the color doesn't "lock in" so you can take a reading, it tends to change shades through a range

#1 Your Salivary Glands have ZERO to do with Acid-Base regulation. Try Kidneys.

Your kidneys are running your body's alkaline status.

And your alkaline status is the secret they don't want you to know.

JPM Oral Hygiene Protocol

This publication is the introduction to JPM. If you paid $2.99 for the kindle version or $4.99 for the paperback version, then you basically paid for the two protocols, the xxxxxxxxxxxxxxxxxx, and the Secret Weapon, xxxxxxxxx gum-line cleaner. You will notice advertising for the other publications. Don't be upset. You got your $3-5 worth. The same cost as for a venti mocha latte, that's long since gone. The information in this publication will be with you for you to use for the rest of your life, every day.

So, why not take the ABC NCD Quiz!

The first half of the book is all about alkalinity. The secret aspect to your health no one, but a few, will talk about. However, no one covers the subject better and more comprehensively than in ABC Water™. The second half is the Number Crunch Diet™. No recipes, but lots of good sound information on diet. You will learn a lot, as no one discusses it the way I do. I brag a bit about the book, because it's really a great book. It's a compilation of nearly 100 books that I've read. But more of a Synergy, a new approach.

The recipes can be found in *12 Changes A Year* and you can see a sample on www.abcwaterandthenumbercrunchdiet.com

The title *Nontoxic Teeth Whitening and Dental Hygiene System* begins with the two chapters you just read, but includes a one-of-a-kind food-grade teeth whitening system, if you feel you need more whitening. It also includes a commentary on fluoride. Wouldn't you like to know if fluoride's something you should be doing, or something you shouldn't be doing?

So put your thinking cap on and let's start the Quiz!

It's good for you!

Pick the correct answers – There may be more than one

1. A urine pH of 5 is telling you
   a. about your blood pressure
   b. that you're tired
   c. about your alkaline reserves
   d. to see a doctor
   e. that you're healthy and fine

2. Urine pH testing is routinely performed by licensed
   a. social workers
   b. clinical laboratory scientists
   c. respiratory therapists
   d. fitness advisors
   e. nurses and doctors

3. The cost of one month of urine pH testing is _____ the cost of open heart surgery (CABG).
   a. 1/10
   b. 1/100
   c. 1/1000
   d. 1/10,000
   e. 1/100,000

4. The opposite of metabolic acid is dietary
   a. phosphates – found in meats and cola drinks
   b. bicarbonate – found in packaged foods
   c. caffeine – found in green tea
   d. bicarbonate – found in fruits and vegetables
   e. bicarbonate – found in oils and fats

5. Information can be of which types
   a. true
   b. incomplete

c. false

d. clouded

e. secret

6. "Natural Flavor" on a food label is
   a. natural flavor extracts from plants and fruit
   b. glutamates, MSG, altered salts
   c. chemicals that make you addicted to the product
   d. generally safe and good for me
   e. not something I need to worry about

7. During World War II, the people who failed to act early
   a. suffered
   b. died
   c. lost everything
   d. became victims
   e. made it through unscathed

8. Compensating means
   a. saving for retirement
   b. eating foods that lift your mood
   c. doing something to mask something
   d. brushing it out of your thoughts
   e. pleasing others and being a do-gooder
   f. all of the above

9. The reason(s) people are fat
   a. they're born that way
   b. they don't make their own meals
   c. hereditary – handed down from your parents
   d. my body just won't lose fat
   e. they don't see the numbers in what they're eating

10. The "Cheat Day" is
    a. a great way to get food cravings satisfied
    b. required to reset my fat-burning hormones
    c. a 2-8 step backwards day
    d. works well for most people long term
    e. is a popular "trick" that you should buy into

ANSWERS

1. A urine pH of 5 is telling you
    a. about your blood pressure – No, but there is a relationship (see Chapter 24)
    b. that you're tired – No, but there is a relationship (see Chapter 20)
    c. about your alkaline reserves – YES! Get to know your alkaline status by reading this book.
    d. to see a doctor – No, but it can lead to that.
    e. that you're healthy and fine – One number tells you little, 35 numbers a week tells you a lot. Get to know your urine pH.

2. Urine pH testing is routinely performed by licensed
    a. social workers – no
    b. clinical laboratory scientists – Yes, 99% of all urine testing is done by a CLS.
    c. respiratory therapists – no
    d. fitness advisors – no
    e. nurses and doctors – Doctors do perform urine tests in their offices, but they are not looking at urine pH with much depth.

3. The cost of one month of urine pH testing is _____ the cost of open heart surgery (CABG)(a bypass, "cabbage").
    a. 1/10 – no
    b. 1/100 – no
    c. 1/1000 – no
    d. 1/10,000 – Yes. You can test all of your urinations for about

$1 a month (see Chapter 11). A cabbage would run you at least $10,000.
e. 1/100,000 – no. But I believe the potential to save yourself $100,000 in medical treatments is very possible.

4. The opposite of metabolic acid is dietary
   a. phosphates – no, phosphates contribute to acidity
   b. bicarbonate – no, bicarbonate yes, but not from packaged foods
   c. caffeine – no, caffeine is a drug, most drugs are acidic
   d. bicarbonate found in fruits and vegetables – Yes!
   e. bicarbonate found in oils and fats – no, oils and fats are not sources of bicarbonate

5. Information can be of which types
   a. true – Yes, this is a bit what your life is all about. Finding the truth about things.
   b. incomplete – aka, partial truths or half truths, aka, "spin". Do you find your head spinning when you go for fancy medical treatments?
   c. false – lies, yes lies. Don't call them untruths. Lies are Lies. When people lie it's your job to call them on it. Otherwise, "ya got no backbone".
   d. clouded – blurry, muddied, confusion. I could write "scientifically" but I would just make you confused and half lost. How does that help you.
   e. secret – Now we're talking. When they say "buy this stock" you've got to be a moron to buy it. The payoffs and the winners are kept secret, shared through word of mouth.

6. "Natural Flavor" on a food label is
   a. natural flavor extracts from plants and fruit – Well, they would like you to think that, but that's far from reality.
   b. glutamates, MSG, altered salts – Yes, often this is the case.
   c. chemicals that make you addicted to the product – Yes

Absolutely
d. generally safe and good for me – don't buy that line
e. not something I need to worry about – you make your own
choices in life

7. During World War II, the people that failed to act early
Referring to this is grim and bleak. But there are people suffering
and dying every day because they failed to act early. You could say
that WWII is still happening all around us in the United States of
America today. My book can help you not to fall victim to this
death and suffering. So that you make it through your life,
unscathed.

8. Compensating means
   a. saving for retirement – no, but I have seen people who are
      just a little too attached to their portfolios, compensating?
   b. eating foods that lift your mood – no, but food is commonly
      used to compensate
   c. doing something to mask something – Ah-Ha, Yes.
   d. brushing it out of your thoughts – no. It's okay and healthy to
      let go of thoughts, just be sure you're not avoiding your
      issues.
   e. people pleasing – reward seekers may be compensating
   f. all of the above – no, just C. Go back and read C again.

9. The reason(s) people are fat
   a. they're born that way – don't give me that
   b. they don't make their own meals – Bingo! This is key.
   c. heredity – your fat jeans are because of your fat genes – no I
      don't think so
   d. my body just won't lose fat – I hear you. There is not a lot of
      good help out there. Luckily, you've found the right place.
   e. they don't see the numbers in what they're eating – Yes. And
      person D above just needs to look at food mathematically
      (and read the book).

10. The "Cheat Day" is
    a. a great way to get food cravings satisfied – Wrong. I'm a testimony of getting rid of food cravings. See Chapter 38, 39, 40, 41.
    b. required to reset my fat-burning hormones – Wrong. If you get your macros right, your hormones will cooperate just fine.
    c. a 2-8 step backwards day – On page 84 of *The Four Hour Body* the person states that he gains 4.4 lbs on his cheat day. Then he loses it. Can you say "moody"?
    d. works well for most people long term – After reading dozens of diet books, I could not find one that worked long term, so I made my own. It's called the Number Crunch Diet.
    e. a popular "trick" that you should buy into – The Number Crunch Diet isn't about cheating. Although it's full of useful "tricks" that I came up with and use daily.

    You'll be miles ahead of the average person after a while.

Follow-up

Lately I've been doing a lot of proofing of my books, yes, I am the editor and proofreader of my own books. It's intense. More than 1000 pages total. So I have pulled out some of the RYV exercise tools, ("3 cups" and "string beads"). I'm not going to explain them as they are copyrighted by someone else, but I will say that the "3 cups" exercise is really good and helps to relieve fatigue and sharpen your vision. "String Beads" is my second favorite, and you can likely guess how it's done. But this next one is my own.

Go to the Party Store and in the pirate section, buy a couple of eye patches. Keep one in your car, one at your desk, one in the kitchen, and just put it on at some point during your day. I set a timer for 15 minutes. So I will put it over my left eye and hit the timer. When it beeps, I switch eyes and hit the timer again, 15 & 15, 30 minutes a day.

My left eye is great for reading, but not that great for distances. My right eye is the exact opposite, great for distances, but not that great for reading. So, with my left eye covered, I do desk work (close-up work), and I force my right eye to work harder and to see close up. Then at 15 minutes I switch sides and cover the right eye, and I do yardwork or household chores (distance work), and force my left eye to see far away.

When the 30 minutes are completed, I go back to using both eyes, and it's amazing how much clearer and less straining and fresher my vision is.

So add in this exercise. And again, who cares what people think if they see you pulling weeds in your backyard with an eye patch on. Orlin was very much against wearing glasses, he encouraged people to fight for their vision and work their eyes, rather than resorting to the quick fix and putting on a pair of glasses.

Use the VIP for outer-eye strengthening and stretching (plus the night vision and pirate exercises), and the RYV for ocular muscles.

www.ingramcontent.com/pod-product-compliance
Lightning Source LLC
Chambersburg PA
CBHW070244290526
45789CB00004B/1751